Health is Wealth

Health is Wealth

Your Mantra for a Healthy, Successful, and Happy Life

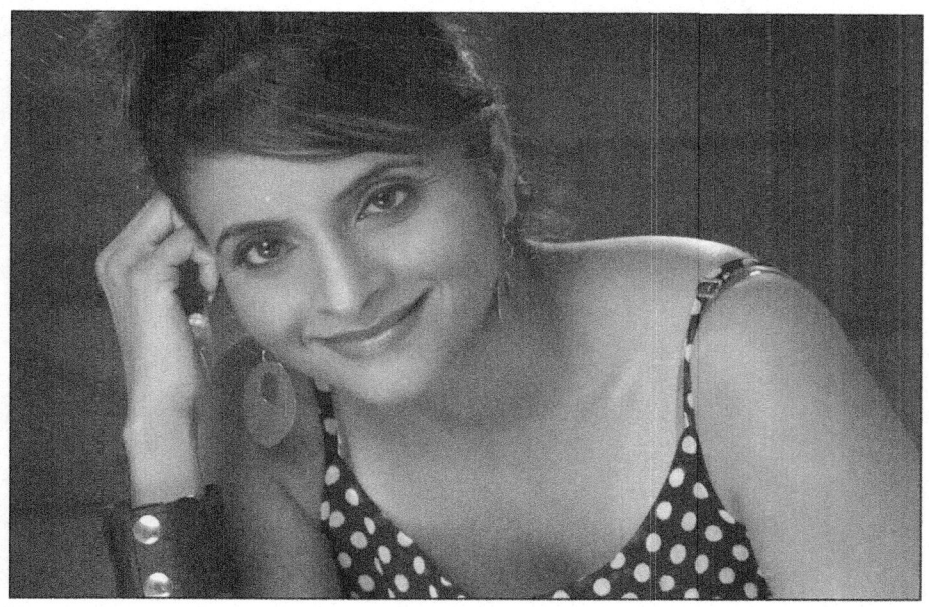

PRIYA CHAVAN

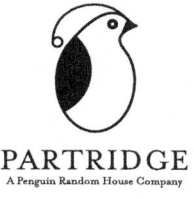

PARTRIDGE
A Penguin Random House Company

Copyright © 2015 by Priya Chavan.

ISBN:	Softcover	978-1-4828-5856-3
	eBook	978-1-4828-5855-6

All rights reserved. No part of this book may be used or reproduced by any means, graphic, electronic, or mechanical, including photocopying, recording, taping or by any information storage retrieval system without the written permission of the author except in the case of brief quotations embodied in critical articles and reviews.

Because of the dynamic nature of the Internet, any web addresses or links contained in this book may have changed since publication and may no longer be valid. The views expressed in this work are solely those of the author and do not necessarily reflect the views of the publisher, and the publisher hereby disclaims any responsibility for them.

Print information available on the last page.

To order additional copies of this book, contact
Partridge India
000 800 10062 62
orders.india@partridgepublishing.com

www.partridgepublishing.com/india

Contents

Introduction vii
1. Good Health 1
2. Maintaining Good Health 5
3. Exercise 6
4. Yoga 8
5. Dance as a Form of Fitness 11
6. Sports/Games for Fitness 13
7. Swimming as a Fitness Form 15
8. Walking/Running/Jogging/Marathons 16
9. Spinning/Cycling as Fitness Activities 17
10. Martial Arts 18
11. Weight Training 19
12. Trekking 20
13. Meditation 22
14. Sleep as a Stress Buster 25
15. Laughter as a Stress Buster 27
16. Relaxation/Massages/Spas 28
17. Nutrition 30
18. Law of Attraction 42

About the Author 45

Introduction

How did I get introduced to this wonderful world of fitness and wellness? Was I born healthy or a fitness lover? No, my dear friends. I was born just like you in a normal, middle-class, Maharashtrian family from Mumbai, India, who believed in academics.

We were not food lovers; hence, we always ate in moderation and simple home-cooked food. We were never into fitness at all. Nor were we encouraged into it or in sports.

I was a scholarly student heavily into academics since childhood. I hated food. Eating was a big torture for me. I remember my mother sitting next to me at the dinner table when I was a child with a stick in her hand and forcing me to eat vegetables or otherwise she would spank me.

I never ate any vegetables or nutritious food. I was thin like a skeleton, very weak, not into any sports activities. I was a nerd and a bookworm.

Although I was a super successful in my SSC examinations by scoring 89 per cent, I was a total failure when it came to my health. I weighed only thirty-five kilograms at fifteen years old. I was not even close to being called a woman as I looked like a skeleton. No guys ever came to talk to me as I was physically not appealing to them.

I was flat on the front and behind. That was me when I was fifteen years old. The biggest turning point came into my life when I went to college for my eleventh and twelfth standards. Being an academic scholar, I opted for science. I looked around me. There were so many pretty girls of my age who were so well built and grown as a teenager. All the guys in college would flock to them. I had my group of friends, but clearly, I was the odd man out among them as I was too thin and small.

No guy even looked at me as I looked like a small child and not a teenage girl. Although I excelled in my studies, my innermost desire was to be like one of the sexy, hot, gorgeous, attractive college girls in the campus who always had guys around them. I would always compare myself to them physically and wonder why I didn't have their assets. Why was I not able to attract guys like them?

The answer was simple. I really didn't eat at all. Hence, I was not gorgeous like them. Then I took a resolution and decided to eat a lot. I would gorge on like eight to ten chapattis forcibly every day to put on weight to develop my assets and curves.

I was called a minor dinosaur at home. Now my food was being compared to food for six people in the family. Earlier, I used to not even eat my own food completely. Such was my obsession to put on weight. I gradually increased my weight to fifty-two kilograms from thirty-five in two years time. Then I was satisfied. The first important lesson I learned in college was to eat healthy if you want to look good and attractive.

My love for fitness was strengthened due to a stimulus at home. My mother caught diabetes and several other ailments, like high blood pressure, cancer. She underwent several health challenges, medical treatments, operations, doctors, hospitals.

She suffered for almost eight years after her retirement as a principal of a school. Looking at her plight, I realized no matter how much money you spend on doctors and medical treatments, the patient does not get relief. Plus you spend lakhs of rupees on it and top of it so much stress and worry in the family.

I learned my second important lesson. Stay away from diseases, be healthy and fit, and go for prophylaxis treatment (i.e. preventive fitness therapy) to stay away from diseases and to be fit and healthy. From that day onwards, I was very clear that I wanted to stay away from doctors, medicine, hospitals forever and to be fit and healthy forever.

At that time, I was climbing the corporate ladder as a marketing manager in the pharmaceutical industry. For those who are yet to know me, I am a qualified bachelor in pharmacy with an MBA in marketing from Mumbai University. I was following an unhealthy eating pattern. I had put on a lot of weight from fifty to seventy-five kilograms. Everyone was making fun of me. They would comment on me that I looked like an eight-month-pregnant woman. I didn't pay attention to them. But once I saw my own photo, I was ashamed of myself.

Now I decided to hit the gym to lose weight and be healthy. It was a wake-up call for me. That was when my fitness journey started. I joined a gym, hired a personal trainer. Under his guidance, I was exercising daily for one hour, doing weight training and functional training. Additionally, I joined power yoga classes. I was spending a bomb on my fitness. But I knew it was essential.

I changed my food habits. I gave up on junk food and cut off rice, sweets, fried food, fatty food. I ate home food with high nutrient value. Every day I would sweat out in the gym. I lost twenty-five kilograms in a year time due to my efforts. Not only did I become slim and trim, weighing fifty kilograms, but I also realized the additional benefits of exercise and healthy eating.

I looked younger, more beautiful, and had more energy levels than before. I was very happy as endorphins and feel-good hormones were running in my body. My complexion improved, my dark circles vanished, I got my curves, and I began to sleep soundly. Besides these, my productivity in work increased, and my relationships improved as well.

That was when I fell in love with fitness. I knew somewhere in my heart that down the line in life, I am going to do something major in this area. I decided to explore the world of fitness more. I read a lot, attended more seminars/workshops, upgraded my knowledge, and learned a lot. That was how I became a fitness/health/wellness expert.

People don't believe that once upon a time, I was really fat as they look at my current slender, slim frame. It's only when I show my past photo in which I weighed seventy-five kilograms that they believe it. They are amazed at my transformation from a fat, old-looking duckling with dark circles under the eyes into a slender, slim, beautiful, young, bright, dynamic, energetic swan having sharp curves and features with glowing skin and eyes.

Not only have I improved my figure and looks, but also, my productivity in work and my relationships have improved. I am also very happy, positive. People ask me my secret, and I point towards my fitness regimen.

This book is my tribute to all the people in the world who are and who are not fitness lovers. In this, I am sharing lots of secrets of fitness, nutrition, mental health, and physical health.

I am also solving a lot of commonly asked queries and clearing myths and misconceptions on fitness. Lots of doubts are raised when it comes to fitness and nutrition—for example, we should moderately exercise after forty and fifty years of age, ladies should rest when they are menstruating, ladies should exercise less after menopause. These are myths spread by people around us.

Also, many people start working out only when they fall ill and are advised by their doctors to exercise and eat healthy. Most Indians exercise after they touch thirty-five and forty. Till then they have already poisoned their bodies and put on piles of weight and also contracted lifestyle diseases—like diabetes, blood pressure, insomnia, migraine—due to their unhealthy eating habits and improper lifestyle—like eating junk food, fatty food, sweets, alcohol; smoking; having less sleep; being stressed; having long working hours; living a sedentary lifestyle.

My book is an eye-opener for all such people. I want to strongly promote fitness/wellness as a prophylaxis (preventive) treatment and not therapeutic therapy. I strongly recommend fitness to be started at a young age, especially in school and college, and to be made a part of everyday life. Just as you eat and sleep daily, similarly fitness and healthy eating has to be done daily and not once in a blue moon or when you have the time or when you are in a mood to exercise.

Ladies especially approach me to help them lose their weight. Their only concern is to be slim and have a good figure. This is a wrong attitude. I want them to think of fitness not just as a weight loss regimen but as an overall physical and mental activity for overall well-being.

Many girls approach me to lose weight for their weddings. This is a short-term goal. These girls will do anything to lose weight for their D-day. Once they are married, they are back to their normal eating habits. They pile loads of kilograms and become fat. Hence, I strongly recommend, my dear girls, that you do not act on such short-term goals. You will get results, but they will only be short-lived. Hence, have a longer, bigger goal in front of you, like being healthy, fit, disease-free, slim for your entire life even before and after marriage, during pregnancy, after delivery, in middle age, in adulthood, after menopause, after your sixties, etc.

This goal will motivate you to embrace fitness, eating healthy habits for your entire life and for your family. My book will encourage you to broaden your vision for such a noble goal.

Also, my experience has shown that people take fitness very casually and not seriously like the way they take their careers or families. It is the least on their priority list. They will only exercise if they find time after their work. They are not convinced about the benefits of exercise and healthy eating as much as they are of the importance of their work and family.

They will take a break from keeping fit for any stupid reason like being tired, being not in a mood, festivals, guests at home. These same excuses they would never give if they were to work. So I understood they take fitness very casually.

The life of a normal Indian is as follows: he grows up, goes to school/college, starts working, gets married, starts family life. Then after everything is done, somewhere down the line in his late thirties he catches some health problem. He then visits doctors, and now it dawns on him that he has to exercise and eat healthy; otherwise, he will lose his work and family. So he is forced to take up some physical exercises and cut down on junk food and drinking/smoking. But by then, it's already too late. None of these lifestyle diseases can be reversed. Ultimately, he loses his physical and mental health and also lots of money on doctors and medicines. Still, in spite of all this, he is not happy.

My book states that if you want to avoid this situation, then please take fitness and healthy living very seriously, as serious as your career and your family. Don't wait for the disease to strike you. Instead, opt for a prophylaxis lifestyle very early in your life. Make fitness your daily routine and start healthy living as young as you can—in your teens, youth. Out of the twenty-four hours in a day, I am only asking for one hour daily.

My book is about my own journey in the superb world of fitness, with my experiences and stories. All of you can connect to it as I have touched to the grass-roots level—simple language, easy for everyone to follow and understand. I have shared and solved many myths in fitness which an average person has.

If you still have any queries, feel free to contact me. I have given my contact details at the end of the book.

So come and enjoy this journey along with me.

Good Health

What is considered as being in good health?

Why is being healthy important?

These are some questions which many people ask me.

Good health is a combination of being physically, mentally, and spiritually fit. If your energy levels are on the high, you are getting sound and undisturbed sleep for seven to eight hours every night, and if your bowel movement is regular (i.e. in the morning daily), then you are considered fit and healthy.

Being healthy is not being only thin but focusing on overall health. The reasons for being healthy are tremendous.

If you are healthy and fit, then automatically you are more productive in your work and have good relationships. When you are healthy and fit, you tend to take up new challenges both mentally and physically. Exercising releases positive hormones in the body, like endorphins, antidepressants, feel-good chemicals. Hence, you feel very rejuvenated and fresh after a good workout session. You are happy after a good workout.

When you exercise, you feel pain in your body, but once it is done, you tend to loosen up. Your blood flow increases in your body; hence, nutrient supply and oxygen supply increase. Your body's mobility increases; stamina increases.

Many people think that bringing weight under control is the only benefit of exercise. But the benefits are tremendous beyond understanding. Mentally, you are charged after a good workout. You can be very productive; you can fight and win any number of challenges you want.

A person who is healthy, fit is very confident and fearless. He has tremendous power to communicate effectively. Because of the strong flow of positive chemicals in his body, he never cribs or complains but works on solutions. He excels in his work. He grows in his work.

Exercising daily and eating healthy daily can also increase your longevity. Many people argue with me, saying, 'We don't want to live that long. We want to die by eighty years old.' I say, 'Fine, but don't you at least wish to increase the quality of your life?'

Even if you live to eighty years, do you want to have diseases, suffer, give trouble to your children, and be a burden? Plus, on top of it, think of the amount of money you would have to spend on medical treatments, hospitals, doctors. The amount can go up in lakhs of rupees. In spite of spending so much, still you won't get relief from pain and suffering. You will either be living on medicines or on the mercy of your relatives/friends.

Seeing your own pathetic condition, you would compare yourself to the hail, hearty, happy, independent, energetic you in the past. You would go into depression and become irritable, angry, whimsical, snappy. People around would help you to a certain extent, but after that, they would give up and leave you in your condition.

Do you want to suffer like this, or do you want to be full of life, energy, and good health? Do you want to be smiling, positive, independent, and productive, a role model for others? The choice is yours. I have chosen the second option—to be happy and disease-free.

For those who are unaware, exercise prevents ageing. You can look younger, more beautiful, sexier with exercising and eating healthy. That's why all the Hollywood and Bollywood actresses are into fitness and healthy eating—to look younger, more beautiful, sexier, radiant, and glowing.

Perhaps you are unaware that we human beings are supposed to live for 130 years or more. Then why is it that we live on an average of eighty years? The reason is our unhealthy lifestyle. We eat unhealthy food, drink, smoke, have sedentary lifestyles, and have no proper sleep.

And we blame the world, pollution, stress, work pressure, family pressure for it. But it is only we who have to be blamed for it and no one else.

Many people argue with me, saying that they don't have time for exercising or healthy food is expensive. But these same people have time for having fun, watching movies, socializing, partying, clubbing, etc. I'm not saying it is wrong to enjoy and have fun. In fact, I strongly recommend people to enjoy and be happy. But at the same time, I recommend them to also find time to exercise at least for forty-five minutes daily. Am I asking for a lot? Not at all.

Regarding the seconnd thought about fruits and healthy food being expensive, let me tell you that you would be ready to spend on clothes, beauty treatments, cosmetics, restaurants, drinks, jewellery, shoes, bags, spas, massages, etc. The list is long. Yes, I agree that it's very important to have play time and to spend on ourselves, but it is equally important to spend on your health, which includes healthy food like fruits, vegetables, dry fruits, salads, green tea. So you have to have a budget for it every month, the way you have it for your daily necessities.

Many people argue with me, saying that they don't drink or smoke. But there are several loopholes in their eating patterns which they are unaware about. I will discuss this in my chapter on nutrition.

Many people argue with me, saying that they are under a lot of stress, work stress, family problems, etc. But what is stress? I will teach you to deal with stress in my chapter on stress handling.

Ladies especially argue with me, saying that post forty years old, their bodies become rigid, so losing fat is impossible. Post menopause, it's impossible to be fit and have the same energy levels like the way you were in your twenties.

My dear friend, all these are myths. I never argue with them because their minds are blocked. But I just tell them to follow my exercise and diet regimen. I then ask them to evaluate their ideas with the results that I gave them.

Lo and behold, they are excited as it turns out to be that they had misconceptions and wrong beliefs and mental blocks. They were not ready to come out of it by their own selves. Once they started experiencing the benefits themselves, they were convinced.

I know so many ladies in the age group of fifty to sixty-five years who are slim, fit, healthy, beautiful and are very much into fitness.

Many senior-citizen ladies argue with me, saying that they have lived their lives, so now what is the use of being beautiful? Yes, it is important for yourself as you love yourself a lot.

Maintaining Good Health

After understanding why being healthy is important, let's understand in what ways you can maintain good health.

1) Exercise regularly.

2) Eat healthy.

3) Sleep soundly for six to seven hours daily.

4) Think positive.

When I put this across to people, they argue, saying they don't have so much time for doing all this. But, my dear friend, you have to set aside time for all this. All I am asking is only forty-five minutes of daily exercise.

Analyze your day-to-day activities, and cut off time from those activities which consume your time but give you no results. Use that time for your daily exercise and eating healthy patterns.

Exercise

This is a very interesting topic and open for discussion.

Exercise involves any form of physical activity, like running, jogging, swimming, yoga, dancing, aerobics, cycling, spinning, martial arts, kickboxing, weight training, etc. The list is long.

Many teenagers argue with me, saying, 'This is our age for partying, drinking, smoking, clubbing, etc. Exercising is meant to be done after you reach forty years or when you grow old. Till then, you should enjoy.'

Hence, I decided to check on these teenagers. I found them looking much older than their age. Plus, they were devoid of energy. At their tender age, they had so many health problems. In fact, they had aged. They were also not performing in their studies, had several relationship problems with their parents, friends. They were not clear of their goals in life. In short, they were wasting their lives. They were violent, rude, complicated.

On the contrary, I have seen individuals who were in their thirties, forties, fifties and were into fitness religiously who looked much younger than their age, were healthy and fit, were also doing very well in their careers and relationships, and were happy.

Hence, my dear teenage friends, you should start exercising early, especially in your teens. Don't wait for the diseases to strike you and then opt for a healthy lifestyle. Start early in life. Don't wait for a medical calamity to strike you. Teenagers, youngsters, have your fun, but balance it with a healthy lifestyle. Make it a part of your life just like the way you eat and sleep.

See the difference in your life. Your life will change drastically for the better.

Many senior citizens argue with me, saying that gyms are a new concept. In their time, they were non-existent, yet their ancestors were healthy by doing agricultural work and eating three proper meals daily, which were breakfast, lunch, and dinner. So why should they opt for change?

If that were the case, then you wouldn't have opted for all the latest developments in technology—like computers, Internet, smart phones, TVs, cars, social media, etc.—which were non-existent in your fathers' time. You changed because you realized they are for your betterment and growth. Similarly, even when it comes to fitness, you have to accept this as a change for your betterment and growth.

My dear friends, ladies (especially in India) want to be slim and beautiful for their weddings. Hence, they will do anything to lose weight. Once married, they start pigging and putting on weight. Also, after pregnancy, they put on weight. My dear friends, why restrict yourself to such occasions to lose weight? Let it be a permanent affair, lifelong.

I am purposely sharing with you all this because you will also face a lot of such people who will discourage you from exercising and being fit. Just give them a deaf ear. The moment they see the results, they will go to you and ask you the secret of your good health.

Choose any form of exercise which you love because then you will stick to it for a longer time. If you are a sports person, then pursue sports like cricket, badminton, football, swimming. If you are a dancer, then dance as dancing is a very good form of cardiovascular exercise. If you are a yoga person, then do yoga religiously. If you like weights, go for weight training. If you love combination of all, then do all. But do what you like.

Just forty-five minutes daily is more than enough. Many people say, 'We are not from the film industry. We need not have six-pack abs—like Sharukh Khan, Salman Khan, Hrithik Roshan, John Abraham—or hour-glass figures, like Kareena Kapoor or Shilpa Shetty. We don't have to survive on our looks. Hence, we need not spend our time, money, and energy on it.'

I agree, my dear friends. You are right, but I am not telling you to imitate our Bollywood actors or actresses. All I am saying is that you exercise for your health and well-being.

Yoga

I love yoga. I can talk about it for hours, days, months. I am a deep follower of yoga and its teachings. I do yoga for at least four to five times a week for one hour each.

It's an ancient form of exercise originating from India. It's the only form of exercise which works internally and externally. Many people feel it's slow and boring. But many are unaware of its true power and strength.

It's a very ancient form of exercise dating to the days of our epics, like Ramayana and Mahabharata. Yoga is a lifestyle. It is about the asanas, Surya namaskar, pranayama, eating, sleeping, thinking. The teachings of yoga are very powerful.

Most yoga poses are derived from nature. You have Gaumukhasan (cow pose), *garudasana* (eagle pose), *vrikshasan* (tree pose), *natarajasana*, prayer pose, *dhanurasana* (bow-and-arrow pose), *ustrasana* (camel pose), *shashankasana* (rabbit pose), *halasana* (plough pose), *chakrasana* (wheel pose), *bhujangasana* (cobra pose), *mayurasana* (peacock pose), *bhadrasana* (butterfly pose), crow pose, cat pose, and many more. All these asanas improve flexibility and tensility of muscles.

There are a lot of stretching exercises, like forward bends, backward bends, side bends. Yoga believes in synchronization and harmony with nature. Yoga gives lots of emphasis on breathing. This increases oxygen supply to our organs.

There are different forms of yoga—traditional or classical yoga, power yoga, hath yoga, *netra* yoga, hot yoga, aqua yoga, etc.

Yoga helps in anti-ageing, reversing your age, making you look younger, more beautiful, fitter. It builds energy and stamina, improves concentration and brain work. Yoga improves your body posture, self-esteem, skin texture, eyesight. In fact, yoga helps to regulate blood sugar in the case of diabetic patients. It regulates blood pressure. In fact, the benefits are unlimited. Hence, many Bollywood and Hollywood actresses and actors are deeply into yoga.

Yoga also brings peace within oneself. Many people tell me it is slow and boring. It is also very easy. You can watch any you tube video and do it yourself. Agreed, but you need to maintain proper form and posture, which can be done under the guidance of a learned trainer. Also, human beings are lazy. We tend to get into a comfortable position very fast. We release the asana moment since it is painful.

Power yoga is that form of yoga which is more intense. It is the cardio form of yoga, which improves your heart rate and makes you sweat. It was specially designed for losing weight.

The unique thing about yoga is the breathing exercises or pranayama. The meaning is to give life (i.e. prana). These exercises help in regulating your breathing pattern, improving your concentration. Many of my members have told me not to do them and only do asanas and surya namaskar. They feel pranayama is not useful. But actually it's the opposite. Pranayama is more powerful than the asanas and surya namaskar. Hence, it's very important to do them. At least, do so for ten minutes regularly. There are different types of pranayama, like *kapalbhati, anulom vilom, bhastrika*, bhramari, om chanting.

Surya namaskar is a tribute to the sun god. The best time would be early morning as the sun rises. It comprises of ten poses. It is an excellent workout for all the parts of the body. But it's very important to have the proper form for asanas and surya namaskar.

Partner yoga is a very enjoyable form of yoga. Stretches are done with a partner. This helps in synchronization, free flow of energy, and support for each other. Also, it helps in giving and bearing extra pressure which you wouldn't be able to bear alone.

The best time to do yoga is early morning before sunrise or before your day starts. Those who find this difficult can do yoga in the evenings and nights. I strongly recommend that you to take this form of fitness as it will improve your physical and mental strength. Do it for forty-five minutes at least thrice a week.

Your flexibility is increased by holding the poses correctly, in the right form, and for a longer time. Slowly and steadily, you should increase your holding time for each asana from ten counts to one minute, then two minutes, and then three minutes.

Dance as a Form of Fitness

Nothing is more beautiful, invigorating, energetic, stress releasing, and contagious than dance. Earlier, dance was thought of just by those who knew dancing. But ever since it has been promoted as a form of fitness, it has gained popularity. In fact, many of the non dancing crowd have started dancing.

I am a born dancer. I started dancing when I was in school. Then I was put into Kathak, a classical dance, by my mother. I fell in love with Kathak. I finished my Nritya Visharad in Kathak dance from Gandharva Mahavidyalaya. I have been dancing Kathak from the last twenty years. I have done more than 100 shows across India. Later on, I branched into Bollywood, Western dances, Zumba, folk dances, hip hop, salsa, etc.

I cannot tell you how I feel after a good dance session. I go in a different world. I forget all about myself. I go in a trance. I forget my worries, tensions. I am at the seventh heaven of delight.

I am aware of the benefits of dance right from beginning. I feel fresh, my energy levels increase, I feel happy after a good dance session, and I am fit and slim due to dancing. My mental concentration has increased. I know somehow I am going to be a dancer forever. Also, I am disease-free because of dancing.

It's the songs or the music that take you to a different world. You get a kick after a good dance session. You are charged after a good dance workout. That's why people dance when they are happy—to celebrate joy, happiness, victory—as you feel completely free by letting your hair down.

Recently, Zumba as a fitness form has become very popular. To freshers who don't know what Zumba is, it's a dance from Latin America. I am regularly into Zumba myself, and I love it. I have lost tremendous weight due to it.

You can in fact also lose weight. Getting inspiration from Zumba, lots of new dance forms have evolved as a fitness form and are gaining popularity. More and more people are enjoying it tremendously. A fusion of the dance forms Zumba, Bollywood, Western dances, hip hop, salsa, bhangra, folk dance, Tollywood (South), Hollywood, aerobics are available for fitness.

The real reason why members are flocking towards them is the fun and excitement. Hence, they don't get bored, which they would otherwise get in a gym or while doing the monotonous treadmill. Especially for ladies who are least into weight training, Zumba and other dance forms are an excellent option.

Different songs, different dances add variety and remove lethargy. There is no monotony. You don't realize you are actually exercising. You feel you are dancing to the music. The entire environment is very encouraging and motivating. Members gyrate their bodies to the trainer's instructions. It's like you are in a discotheque or a club and not in a gym.

The reason why I am so in for this form of workout is that I really want to help those people who want a healthy alternative to weight training. Also, please, even non-dancers can attend this fitness class. Due to this, dance has gathered the attention of a very big audience.

I strongly recommend this form of workout. Many members tell me that this workout is for young people. But, friends, again this is a myth as people of any age group can do it. In fact, many senior citizens enjoy this workout freely. So, friends, put on your dance shoes and hit the dance floor.

Sports/Games for Fitness

All of you who are sports lovers, please pursue some sport or game of your choice. Outdoor games include cricket, badminton, tennis, football, swimming, basketball, volleyball, kabaddi, hockey; the list is endless.

India is not a sports nation. The only game which is popular here is cricket. Only in this game can you think of pursuing a career and earning money. In developed countries like USA, United Kingdom, and Australia, sports is a very lucrative career. Youngsters are encouraged to pursue different sports. They have good careers in it.

Indians are hypocritical. They feel that playing sports is to be done only during your school days. As you grow old, you should give it up. You should only focus on your career and family. In fact, they make fun of those who enjoy a good game on Sundays or other days.

This is absolutely not true. Please don't listen to such crap. In fact, when you are actively building your career and family, you should devote some time for your favourite sport. At least, play some game. Be a child again. In fact, your muscles and bones become stronger. You are more equipped to handle your work and family pressure effectively. Plus, the joy and pleasure of playing the game of your interest is different. Hence, to all our sports lovers, please pursue a sport/game of your choice irrespective of your age and how busy you are.

Don't be bothered by what others think of you. In fact, you be a role model for others. After seeing you so happily playing, many of your ailing, complaining friends/relatives or agony aunts will follow you.

Many people complain that they want to play but that they don't have a team, group, or place to play. For them, let me tell you there are several groups available who are actively into games. Be a member of such groups. Also, there are many clubs and sports complexes who offer playgrounds, lawns, tennis lawns, badminton courts, swimming pools, table tennis courts, squash court, etc. along with coaches.

You be a member of such sports complexes/clubs and avail of their facilities. Again, some people crib that they cannot afford to pay membership fees of such clubs/complexes. You can take membership from government sports complexes, which are very economic.

Also, if you are fortunate to have a beach near your house, make use of it to pursue your sports. So, friends, gear up, put on your sports shoes, pick up your rackets, run towards the ground for a gruelling game, and enjoy it too. This applies to dear ladies too.

Swimming as a Fitness Form

It is a full-body cardio workout. It is refreshing and invigorating. The feel of water is great. It's extremely enjoyable. Those who are water babies, please pursue this sport.

The only reason why I am discussing so many different forms of fitness is because I have myself experimented with almost all forms of workouts and then zeroed in on those I enjoy and like. Of course, you cannot do all of them. You may not like many of them as well; you will not have that much time.

The whole idea is to pick a workout which you enjoy. A swimming person may not be a dancer or vice versa. It's perfectly fine as long as you do what you like.

Also, don't force yourself into doing a workout which you don't enjoy as you will not stick to it for long. That's why I recommend pursuing what you enjoy.

Also, some people make mistakes by doing only cardio workouts, like sports and dancing. I strongly suggest going for a balance and a mix of cardio, yoga, muscle training along with nutritious diet. This will remove monotony as well as give you variety. Also, you get better and faster results in terms of weight loss and overall fitness.

Walking/Running/Jogging/Marathons

This involves walking/running on a treadmill or in the open in gardens, beaches, parks. It's a very good sport as it involves good cardio activity. Indoor running on a treadmill is also good. A treadmill has several speed options and different inclinations. In fact, it also indicates how much calories you have burned.

Choose a time which suits you the most—morning or evening. At least, walk/jog for forty-five minutes daily or at least thrice a week.

Marathons are becoming popular and spreading like wildfire. People flaunt that they have run marathons. It is a very addictive sport and a good one.

In fact, there are many organizations that encourage participation in marathons. They're also very good networking grounds. Many big celebrities are into marathons.

Spinning/Cycling as Fitness Activities

Do you remember as a child when you were learning cycling? You fell, faltered, or even broke your bones. But ultimately, you learned it. Cycling is an amazing exercise. If you cycle in the open air, it's a beautiful experience.

Spinning is indoor cycling. Many gyms have this as a group activity class. In order to make it exciting, it's done with music and songs from Hollywood, Bollywood, etc.

The trainer gives instructions to increase resistance, go slow or pedal fast, go up and down, take different positions. Songs and loud music add flavour to the entire workout. Many people enjoy this workout.

So, friends, if you are a cycling fan, do try this workout.

Martial Arts

Another good form of work out is martial arts. That's why kick-boxing, karate, military boot camps have become very popular as workouts.

These workouts are very effective in losing weight and toning the body. I am heavily into kick-boxing. I love it. It has given me tremendous results.

It's a myth that these are meant only for men. I, as a girl, am a tremendous kick-boxer, almost hitting 800 kicks on a sandbag at one go in an hour. I imagine someone I hate as the sandbag. I would remove my frustration on it by kicking it hard. I got tremendous results by it. My waist has gone down. My weight has reduced.

There are different types of kicks—front kicks, side ones, back ones, on a stepper, hand kicks, etc. In fact, it's fun.

Ladies, I strongly recommend that you go for this workout form.

Weight Training

Many people feel this is a male domain. If you do this, you will become like a man, muscular. In fact, weight training helps in building muscles. Ladies, this is very important. Once you lose weight and arrive at your standard height-and-body-weight ratio, it's time to build muscles. If you do excessively cardio workouts, you will lose muscles. This can lead to weakness, fatigue, and lethargy. Hence, it is essential to build muscles.

Along with cardio workouts, do weight training for at least thrice a week for at least thirty minutes each.

Ladies, initially you may find it boring, but later on, you will start enjoying it. I strongly recommend it to be a part of your exercise regimen.

Plenty of weight training machines are available for the upper body, lower body, chest, abs, etc. You can increase the intensity of the workout by increasing weights and the number of repetitions gradually.

Initially, to get accustomed to it and to do it correctly, you should do it under a trainer. Once you are thorough with it, then you can do it yourself. Most of the men are very fond of it as it helps them look masculine. Hence, they are highly motivated.

I have encountered many women who are into weight training a lot. They have toned bodies.

Trekking

Can trekking be categorized as a workout? Yes, very much. I was never a trekker. But I used to hear wonderful stories of trekking from my friends who were avid trekkers.

They would tell me it's addictive. I never knew its value until I went for a nature trek through my gym. In fact, I was not ready, but my trainer pursued me a lot and finally convinced me to go for it. Thanks to him, I enjoyed it a lot. It was a mountain trek. In the midst of nature, we went up the mountain. It was an excellent workout, full of energy. We created a new group that was into health and fitness.

Trekking is advisable in monsoons and winter season, but not summer as its very hot. Plenty of trekking groups are available on the Net. You can contact them and be one of them.

Let me take a break and ask you guys how you find the journey so far. Does it sound like an exercise manual? Does it sound boring and informative? You might say, 'We already know all this. Is there anything else you can offer besides this?'

You may say that you can google all this information. I agree; you are right. But what sets me apart is that I have experience. Whatever I have shared with you till now is from my experience, not theory.

Lot of books are also available. You can read them and be well versed with them. But I am providing you with real, live experiences of mine and others. What I have shared with you are true, honest, real facts and not hypothetical ones.

The constant challenges one faces are common ones, which you will also face and endure. They cannot be shared by a book or Google. I motivate you to make fitness a part of your life unlike books/Google, which are just information providers.

I share with you success stories of ordinary people, not extraordinary ones, with whom you can connect and achieve your goal.

Hence, my book is different. There are millions of people on this earth to whom fitness is last on their to-do list. It's a challenge to convince them. My book is for them. Also, I have not projected fitness as some sort of punishment but a wonderful, beneficial regimen.

For those who are convinced on fitness but not doing anything about it, I have taken them a step further. By reading my book, they will be charged and will start their fitness regimen.

For those who are already into fitness, I have showed them to explore different avenues in fitness. I have undergone each and every thing I have discussed. That's why I can confidently talk about them.

Meditation

After discussing physical workouts, let's go to mental workouts. Is it important to do them? What are they? Are they effective? Do they really exist? Are they just something? Aren't you exercising your mind when you are doing physical exercises? And so many questions are asked.

Yes, first of all, mental exercises are equally important like physical ones. In yoga, you are exercising your mind along with your body.

In fact, in all exercise forms—be it dancing, martial arts, sports, games, swimming—your mind is getting exercised simultaneously as you have to concentrate to do them correctly and excel in them. But there are some special mental exercises which are only meant for the brain.

Meditation is an exercise to improve mental strength. Many people think it's so simple to meditate—just sit in one place with your eyes closed. Try doing it yourself; you would not be able to sit still in one place for even a minute. The reason is you will be distracted by many thoughts, personal and professional, and the very purpose of meditation is lost.

There are different types of meditation—viz. vipassana, Brahmavidya, Greek, candle gazing. Should you know all this? Not really, as long as you meditate in some form or other. Vipassana meditation is from Gautama Buddha. Plenty of vipassana centres are there in India. Plenty of CDs are available.

Through this, you focus on your inner self as you go deep within yourself. You discover yourself.

Brahmavidya meditation is a very powerful one. It is an extension of yoga. It focuses on loving yourself the most on this earth. In fact, yoga also preaches the same thing. It says that every morning, you get up and say in front of the mirror 'I am the best', 'I love myself the most', 'I am the most healthy person on this earth', 'I am the strongest', 'I am desirable', etc.

By this, you are increasing your self-worth. You are building strength within yourself. You become unstoppable. You become powerful, independent. Nobody on this earth can challenge you. No matter the problem, you will face it and solve it.

You must meditate compulsorily for fifteen minutes daily. Many people tell me, 'You are telling us to exercise, eat healthy, and also meditate now. With so much to be done, we would end up only doing this the entire day. So when will we work, earn money, take care of our families?' That's why, my dear friends, one must plan one's day.

All I am asking is forty-five minutes of your precious time daily and fifteen minutes of meditation daily. Is this a lot? Anyway, you do spend time watching movies, TV, socializing, etc. Can't you spare one hour daily out of the twenty-four hours? If not every day, then at least three times a week.

Nothing is impossible if you decide to do it. It's for your health. You would save lakhs of rupees which otherwise you would have spend on medical treatments, doctors, hospitals, medicines later on in life due to illness.

You may argue that's a fact of old age, that nobody can escape from it. This is a myth. It's not necessary that in old age you have to undergo health challenges. If you take care of your health, eat healthy, exercise, sleep well, and avoid stress, you can retard several so-called health challenges. Anyway, what is old age? Who decides what is old? Age is just a number. Read Deepak Chopra's book *Ageless Body, Timeless Mind*.

Ideally, we human beings are supposed to live for 130 years or more. But we end up living for only an average of eighty years. Have you ever analyzed why? You would say that's the truth and that we cannot change this fact of life. We live only so few years because of our lifestyle. We eat unhealthy food, like junk food, sweets, fried food, spicy food. We drink, smoke. We are lazy, don't exercise, lead a sedentary lifestyle. We don't sleep well. We take lots of stress. All these poison our bodies; we start deteriorating at a faster pace than we are supposed to do.

Yes, we should enjoy good food, but do it in moderation and occasionally. Enjoy your drinks, again within control. Be ambitious but work with a balance of play and family so that stress does not catch you. Lot of things are beyond your control. You wouldn't have known so many things till I have told you about it. But you can control at least which is within your frame. Instead of worrying over a problem, you can work towards a solution. When you go to sleep, forget everything that happened in the day and sleep well. We normally hold on to negative memories but never become happy by remembering our good work. The list is long enough.

That's what causes stress. Remember the good things which give you pleasure. Laugh. Be a child. Do things which give you pleasure.

That's why, friends, you can retard your old age also. It's in your hands. Ladies, you can retard menopause also. You will look younger, your wrinkles will vanish, and your complexion will glow.

Do it and see for yourself.

Sleep as a Stress Buster

Many people in India feel guilty if they sleep peacefully and well. In fact, they feel proud and flaunt proudly that yesterday they slept only for four hours. Whether you were working or partying, that's immaterial. Then to make up for the loss of sleep, they end up sleeping late in the morning hours. This destroys their body cycle, and they fall ill.

Many argue, saying that in their jobs or work, there are no proper hours of working, late-night shifts, etc. I agree certain things are beyond your control, but at least, when you have late-night shifts, then regularize your sleeping pattern.

Ideally, you should have seven to eight hours of sound and undisturbed sleep daily. Sleep early, and rise early. The age-old adage 'Early to bed and early to rise makes a man healthy, wealthy, and wise' is 100 per cent true. Don't drink beverages like tea or coffee before going to bed as it will keep you awake.

Why you should sleep well at night? The reason is the body needs rest after a day's hard work. Also, new cells are generated when you are asleep. You feel fresh and rejuvenated after a good night's sleep. The body is like a machine. It also needs oiling and rest time and again. Sleeping provides rest to the body.

Plan your day in such a way that you hit the pillow by at least 11 or 12 p.m. Manage your work in such a way that this is achieved. Sleep well at night and be up by 6 a.m. at least. Do your one-hour of exercise and meditation daily.

If you are unable to do it, then do it in the evening or night. But do it compulsorily. If you are having a late party or a night out or social gathering, see that you restrain yourself to doing it only once or twice a week. Or see to it that you don't make it a regular habit as slowly and steadily it will start affecting your health negatively. You become weak, start sagging, develop black circles under your eyes, and look older than your age. If socializing is due to work commitments, then see to it that you don't stay out late for long. Everything comes with practice.

Laughter as a Stress Buster

Have you ever noticed that people who laugh a lot are also very healthy, whereas those who are anxious, depressed, constantly worrying, cribbing, complaining are suffering from stress-related disorders, like high blood pressure, diabetes, ulcers, gastric disorders, migraine, insomnia, or sleeping disorders? They are also irritable. They are obese and look older than their age.

What do I mean by older than your age? This means that your biological age may be twenty-five years but your internal organs would be like those of a sixty-year-old, which are deteriorated to that extent in terms of functioning. So if you can age faster, then you can also retard your age.

Hence, laughter is the best medicine. Be happy with what you have and work towards more. Laugh over your own mistakes. Laugh like a child. Don't be stern with a straight face. Smile a lot. Those who are serious can join laughter clubs. There they make you compulsorily laugh loudly. Watch comedy movies, shows, crack jokes, forgive yourself for mistakes, move on, and love yourself.

Laughter releases all the negative energy from your body. It boosts the flow of positive, healthy chemicals in your body. It makes you feel good, powerful, energetic. Hence, friends, start laughing a lot.

Relaxation/Massages/Spas

In India, people are not accustomed to holidays. They feel guilty if they enjoy feeling happy. They feel if they are working, they have to be stressed up. This is a wrong notion. Abroad—especially Americans, Europeans, Australians—people believe in enjoying life. They maintain a good balance between work and play.

When they work, they really work. They don't waste time. When they play, they play hard. They have a tradition to enjoy their weekends by going to another place, beaches, resorts, another country. When they enjoy, they cut themselves away from the entire world. They only enjoy and relax. In India, even if our people go on a vacation, their work and other problems will tag along with them. End result, they don't achieve anything. Neither are they able to enjoy fully nor are they able to work properly. They sit on the fence, not knowing where to jump.

As a result, they come back more tired from a vacation. That's why, my friends, it's very important to enjoy fully.

It's very important to have play time and me time, where you let your hair down and enjoy, relax thoroughly, as this charges your battery and you feel rejuvenated. So, friends, balance your time. Work for eight to nine hours daily. In the remaining time, do your exercise, pursue your hobbies, enjoy with your friends and family. The key to happiness and success is balancing your life. You would say: 'It is easier said than done', 'My boss is very strict, he does not allow me to leave the office before 9 p.m.', 'I have deadly targets', 'I am barely able to spend time with my family, how will I set aside time for exercise and hobbies?'

My dear friends, everything is possible if you have a strong willpower. Devote Sundays only for yourself and family and friends. Enjoy. Do things that you like—e.g. watch a movie, have lunch or dinner out, socialize, attend good motivational seminars/workshops, be a part of a club/group/team, take rest, sleep, go out on a vacation, go for shopping (especially the ladies), go to a spa, have massages.

It's very important to take these breaks and relax and chill as this charges your battery. You will again be empowered to go back to work. You will perform better as you are happy unlike those who just drag themselves to work as they are not happy.

Your relationships will also improve as you have happy hormones running in your body. You will stop feeling frustrated, irritable and will start accepting, avoiding stress.

That's why people who live balanced lifestyles are also very successful in their lives professionally and personally; this is a proven fact. Those who overdo something are unhappy and lead a mediocre life. I agree that even they live life, but see the quality. Is this something you want? Or do you want to achieve your goals and be happy as well?

Benefits of Massages

Massages increase blood flow. This means that there is increase in nutrients and oxygen. Blood is the main carrier of nutrients and oxygen. That's why, after a good massage, you feel relaxed and happy and your skin glows.

If possible, then do take them as far as possible, considering your budget and time.

Nutrition

This is a very, very, very important topic. You are what you eat. Besides being a qualified bachelor in pharmacy and having an MBA, I am also a nutritionist.

Besides having technical knowledge about it, I also have practical knowledge. As I shared with you, I was very fat once upon a time, weighing seventy-five kilograms for a frame of five feet three inches.

With determination, I lost twenty-five kilograms in a year's time, almost two kilograms per month. Now I weigh forty-six kilograms. The biggest role was played by my diet. I also exercised a lot, including a combination of workouts like kick-boxing, functional training, dancing, power yoga.

So many people are not aware that 90 per cent of weight loss is due to diet control. They exercise a lot and then go home and eat everything and anything on this earth. Then they put on calories and complain why they are not losing weight. Let me tell you, my friends, you have to combine your exercise with proper diet.

Several myths exist about diet, one of them is that dieting means not eating anything at all. That's why people are scared of dieting. I correct them, telling them that dieting means eating the correct nutritious food at the correct time.

The following are some misconceptions about dieting:

- 'What is the correct food? You mean to say we don't eat healthy? In fact, my wife and mother are experts in nutrition. They know the best.'

- 'I am not fat. I am chubby cute. I have been like this since childhood. I have a tendency to put on weight. My body's metabolism is slow. Hence, I put on weight fast and cannot lose fast.'

- 'I am over forty years old. Now I cannot change my diet. If I go on a diet, I feel weak, giddy. My work requires a lot of energy. Hence, I need to eat well to cope with the work pressure, stress.'

- 'I travel a lot in my work. I have no choice but to eat outside food. I have social commitments. Hence, I cannot say no to food and drinks; otherwise, I will not be accepted socially.'

- 'I am a foodie. I love food. I cannot give up my favourite items. We live to eat. We work for what? For only living and eating.'

So on and so forth the list of misconceptions continues. These are misconceptions which people have developed due to their imagination and due to listening to other people.

First of all, dieting doesn't mean not eating anything at all. It means eating the right food at the right time.

What is right food? It is a balanced diet, which comprises of a combination of carbohydrates, proteins, vitamins, minerals, nutrients, and fats.

So where do we get them from? Wheat and rice are good sources of carbohydrates. Carbohydrates provide energy. Proteins help in building muscles. Vitamins, minerals, nutrients are important for providing energy, strength, and stamina to the body.

Everything has a role to play. Hence, I recommend a balanced diet. But we Indians are fond of carbohydrates. In the North, a lot of wheat is consumed, and in the South, rice is consumed. Instead of depending on your lifestyle, you have to consume carbohydrates. If you lead a physically active life, then you need more energy. Hence, you need to consume more carbohydrates to burn more calories.

If you lead a sedentary lifestyle, like an office job or stay-at-home job, then consume less carbohydrates. Hence, it's very important to consume food depending on your lifestyle.

However, in both cases, you should consume more proteins, vitamins, minerals, and nutrients in your food.

Pulses, sprouts, various types of dal, chana, soybeans are the best sources of vegetarian proteins. The non-vegeterian sources are fish, chicken, egg whites. Vegetarians normally complain of being deficient in proteins, but they can compensate by consuming the vegetarian sources. Also, egg whites can be consumed.

Fruits, vegetables, salads are the best sources of vitamins, minerals, and nutrients. And surprisingly, people hate them the most. I don't advocate vegetarianism, but I do strongly recommend increasing consumption of vegetables in your day-to-day diet.

Here, again people have wrong ideas. They eat only those vegetables which they like. This is comfort zone. In fact, when I was in school and college, when I did not know about nutrition, I used to eat only potatoes, a few pulses, eggs, chicken, and fish. I would avoid other vegetables and fruits.

Also, people have a liking for a particular fruit or vegetable. They ensure that they eat those as many times as possible in the week. This is a wrong practice because that vegetable and fruit has limited nutrients. You would be deficient in other vitamins. Hence, go for different variety of foods daily.

All the mothers in the world, I pay respect to them as they feed their families. But there are certain things which you should also know about nutrition.

Firstly, there is something called RDA, which is recommended daily allowance. Our body requires carbohydrates, proteins, vitamins, minerals, nutrients. You need to consume the right amount of nutrients every day according to your RDA. We Indians have a tendency to eat more carbohydrates in the form of chapattis, rice, bread. We don't eat proteins adequately nor vitamins, minerals, and nutrients.

Human beings are supposed to be vegetarians. Our small intestines are very long, like that of a vegetarian animal (elephant, deer, rabbit, cow). We don't have long sharp canine teeth like carnivorous animals (tigers, lions, etc.), who feed on flesh. They require sharp teeth to tear the flesh. So we are actually going against the law of nature.

But I have no hard feelings for those who are non-vegetarians. In fact, I advocate fish and chicken as ideal sources of proteins as they have high amounts of it.

But my only advice is to increase intake of vegetables, fruits, salads, proteins, and organic food in your diet rather than just stuffing yourself with carbohydrates.

Carbohydrates like rice, chapattis, and bread provide energy to the body. So eat less of them. Eat them based on your lifestyle's energy requirement. If your lifestyle demands lots of physical work, then have high amounts of carbohydrates. If you lead a sedentary lifestyle (desk job), then consume less.

Also, compulsorily have in your diet proteins like eggs, sprouts, dal, pulses, chicken, fish.

Vitamins form a very important component. There are different types of vitamins, like A, B, C, D, E, K. Out of them, vitamins A, D, E, and K are oil-soluble ones. The rest are water-soluble ones. The biggest source of vitamins are fruits and vegetables.

That's why consume daily at least portions of two different vegetables. Do not repeat the same vegetables. Go for different vegetables daily. Many people are very selective in choosing vegetables. They eat only those they like. This is not correct. You should eat different vegetables daily as every vegetable has different vitamins and minerals. As told to you earlier, the body requires all of them for proper functioning. For example, if you eat cabbage and brinjal today, then tomorrow eat spinach and lady's finger, and then on the third day different vegetables.

Same is the case with fruits. We should eat at least three different fruits daily. Also, eat different fruits daily. Don't repeat them. For example, if today you eat banana, apple, and orange, then tomorrow you eat something different, like watermelon, berries, *chikoos*; on the third day, again eat different fruits from the first two days, like grapes, sweet lime, guava. This is just an example. You can eat seasonal fruits.

Many people will argue with me and say, 'What you are advising is not practical. If we only cook healthy food, then nobody in the family likes it, and then ultimately, we'll have to finish them. Ladies especially complain that their children and their husbands love tasty food and are not into nutritious food at all.

Fruits rich in vitamin C, like citrus fruits (oranges, sweet lime), helps in anti-ageing, makes your skin look healthy, young, and glowing. Berries like strawberries and blueberries are rich in antioxidants. They help you to prevent ageing and give you a younger, wonderful skin.

Bananas are rich in iron. Cucumber provides cooling, gets rid of dark circles below your eyes. Hence, in beauty parlours, they put pieces of cucumber on the eyes to make the eyes look fresh and get rid of dark circles.

Carrots are rich in vitamin A. They help to make your eyes healthy. Beet root and leafy vegetables are rich in iron. It helps to improve blood flow.

Among dry fruits, almonds are very healthy. I recommend all my members to eat a handful of dry fruits daily, which are almonds, cashew nuts, walnuts, raisins, dates, pistachios. You can have five to six almonds daily; the rest of the dry fruits, you can have two to three pieces each. Whenever you feel hungry in between meals, instead of binging on junk food, eat a handful of these.

Not only will they satisfy your hunger, but they'll also provide you energy, stamina, and nutrition. Almonds are rich in omega-3 fatty acids, which are important for the hair, skin, brain, and heart. They improve concentration, memory, and stamina.

Walnuts are also rich in omega-3 fatty acids.

But as leaders, financial managers, and nutritionists of the house, my dear friends, ladies, you have to take the lead in convincing your families to this lifestyle. You have to convince them on the health benefits and, if need be, force it on them. You should not succumb to them; otherwise, they will dominate you and have their way. When they fall ill due to an unhealthy lifestyle, then you have to take care of them and spend a bomb on doctors and medicines. Is this what you want?

Initially, they may resist, but later on, when they see that their energy levels have increased due to the healthy lifestyle, they will love it and thank you for it. So, my dear friends, don't get bogged down by their comments, and carry on with your good work.

Let me tell you that fruits offer us the most benefits. I was never a fruit lover. But when I got introduced to the wonderful world of yoga, I started attending plenty of workshops. In one of them, I was introduced to sattvic food.

Three types of food are available: sattvic, tamasic, and rajasic. Sattvic is spiritual food. Any food from natural and organic sources is sattvic food, which includes vegetables, fruits, salads, water. Sattvic food gives energy to the body. It detoxifies the body. It is rich in nutrition, less in calories.

In fact, one needs to drink a minimum of three to four litres of water daily. Our body is 70 per cent water. Most of us drink only one to two litres daily. Try eating more raw food.

This is wrong as water helps in detoxification and brings glow to the face. Your skin looks fresh and nice. Also, less water in the body leads to dehydration. Ladies, drink at least two to three litres daily and, gentlemen, three to four litres daily. Water also helps in digestion and helps in maintaining the body's pH balance.

Tamasic food gives heat to the body, like non-vegetarian food, meat, alcohol, spicy and masala food, cigarettes. It makes you angry, violent, aggressive in a wrong way. In fact, it triggers a lot of negative and violent emotions.

Rajasic food is oily and heavy, like fried food and sweets. It makes you put on weight and makes you drowsy, less active; it has less nutrient value and more calories.

Consume more of sattvic food in your diet. You can occasionally consume tamasic and rajasic food if you cannot resist them. But most of the people do the reverse. They have more of tamasic and rajasic food in their diet. On certain occasions—like festivals, social gatherings, parties—you can enjoy them. But immediately burn the excess calories by exercising, and balance it with sattvic food the next day. In this way, you can prevent piling weight.

But, my friends, what you do is relish that food for days together, not burn the excess calories, and hardly eat sattvic food. Then you complain of being fat, lethargic, drowsy, lacking energy, suffering from gastrointestinal disorders, like indigestion, heart problems. Oily food triggers cardiovascular problems, headaches, sagging, dull skin, black circles under the eyes, fast ageing, hair fall, dull hair, coughing, sleep disorders, stress, etc.

You are the cause of your problems. Do you know that research has found out that 70 per cent of doctors' patients are suffering from stress-related disorders? What is stress? It is caused due to your unhealthy lifestyle.

Nowadays, people have many challenges—career, relationship, monetary problems, spiritual needs. I empathize with them. In order to deal with them, they follow a loop. Either they drink, smoke, dope, or have sex for stress relief.

But these methods provide only a temporary solution. They never get rid of the real cause. In fact, they cause more deadly side effects. Addiction and dependence are few of them. Plus, you have a hangover the next day, not to mention the guilty feeling which accompanies them. So weekends they party and indulge in all this for stress relief. For the time being, they forget their worries. Again, on Monday they are back to the real world, where the challenges are waiting for them.

They feel weak and dependent, have a hangover, and cannot face them. Again, they try to escape by turning to alcohol. Their productivity in work goes down, and their relationships suffer as they are depressed and unhappy. Their health suffers.

Hence, this is a vicious cycle. Every weekend, they go to it and end up in rehabilitation centres. They look like zombies.

There is nothing wrong in occasional partying and having drinks or smoking. But see that they're under control and manageable. They should not affect you, and you shouldn't be dependent on them either.

We Indians have a tendency to eat a healthy breakfast, a full lunch, and a heavy dinner as normally we have dinner with family. Almost a gap of six to seven hours is maintained in between meals. Then they pig out at meals and complain to have put on weight. In between meals, they satisfy their hunger by binging on junk food (like *vada pav*, samosas, bhelpuri), tea, coffee, biscuits, cigarettes, etc.

It is this consumption of junk food which makes them put on weight. These are the same people who complain that they don't have money to buy fruits as they are expensive. Surprisingly, they have all the money to buy junk food.

As I have stated earlier, you can enjoy tasty junk food but not daily. Eat them on weekends or occasionally to satisfy your taste buds so that you do not have any regrets later on. Eating them daily is what creates a problem.

Whenever you feel hungry in between meals, eat healthy food, like dry fruits, fruits, salads. Consume only one to two cups of tea or coffee daily. This lifestyle I am suggesting generally. It will be more specific and customized as per the need and requirement of the individual, taking into consideration the lifestyle, habits, medical condition, etc.

Many people complain that fruits, vegetables, and water are tasteless. Well, for you, you can make some innovative recipes which will include them and make them tasty as well. If you cannot, then forcibly develop a taste for them. Many people are allergic to them. You can opt for fruit juices if fruits are unpalatable to you.

But ensure that, by hook or crook, you have them in your stomach. Fitness and nutrition is a religion. It has to be followed daily and not intermittently as per your whims and fancies.

I have personally coached lakhs of people for fitness and nutrition through Priya's Wellness Centre. Only 5 per cent are serious about their health. The rest of them only do it to pass time. They do it as a social status symbol, out of boredom as they have nothing else to do, to kill time, or to make friends. It's not that they are poor and cannot afford healthy food. It's just their casual attitude towards their health.

In fact, they justify that life is meant to be lived. Hence, we should enjoy and eat whatever we want to. I try to change this attitude and tell them that in the long run, they will suffer health-wise. They again justify that they will cross the bridge when they get to it. They have enough money to spend on doctors and medicines then. Sure, you must have, but is it worth spending on them? And is there a guarantee that even after spending a bomb on them, you will get relief?

In fact, 99 per cent of such cases don't get relief and are in pain and distress. In fact, they become a burden on themselves and their families. And believe me, the amount of money they spend is actually much more than they had anticipated. In fact, they end up taking loans. Imagine the stress that you and your family will go through.

I will give you an example myself. My mother, after retiring as a principal of a school, suffered from cancer. She underwent chemotherapy and radiation as treatment. After recovering from it, she suffered from spinal problem. She was diagnosed with diabetes and high blood pressure. She is now seventy years old.

She has been still struggling for the last fifteen years. You have no clue how much money was spent in her treatment.

In fact, the best doctors cannot help you. You only have to take care of yourselves. So why go through all this? Instead, start leading a healthy life from an early age. In fact, start moulding your children to a healthy lifestyle rather than to a junk lifestyle.

This is the biggest gift you can give to your child. He will be indebted to you for your entire life. Many teenagers argue with me that in their age, they should enjoy and have fun, eat, drink, binge on junk food, smoke, and dope. Healthy living and eating should be done later in life after forty years of age. This is absolutely wrong. If they follow their current lifestyle, by the time they reach forty years old, they will have aged twice then their actual age, would have contracted all the diseases due to their previous unhealthy lifestyle, would for sure be diabetics or BP patients, and have stress and depression. They would also not be very successful in their work as well as in their relationships as a healthy lifestyle is directly proportional to success in work and relationships. In fact, I know many of my friends who have declined like this.

When they are in their forties, they look as if they are in their fifties. In fact, many forty-year-old with healthy lifestyles have reversed their ages, look in their twenties, and have high energy levels. They are fit, healthy, and super successful in all aspects of their lives.

This is a hard and proven fact. I can prove it to you with this with statistics. Lots of such cases are around me. Hence, teenagers, don't boast of your lifestyle and say that you are the new generation so our thoughts are outdated and old-fashioned.

So, teenagers, youngsters, beware of your lifestyle and reform it ASAP as experience is the best teacher.

Till now, I have shared with you the cases of those who are lazy with their health. But there are also opposite cases of those who are obsessed with their weights. This can also be equally dangerous. In fact, it can be a mental disorder.

This is especially seen in the cases of models, actresses, and people who are glamorous and from the beauty industry. Even if they are slim, they want to be thinner. They want a perfect body, face, and body statistics. They are always discussing these with their friends as if these are the only important things in life.

Let me tell you, my friends, you can never be perfect. Accept yourself the way you are, and love yourself they way you are. Aim towards being healthy. Even if you are a few kilograms up and down, its fine. Focus on your skills, intellect, personality, communication, and talent, not just on external beauty. You should be smart. Ultimately, in the long run, all these count and matter.

Those who are looking for weight loss, try eating small meals after every two hours. Your dinner should be light. Follow the saying 'Eat breakfast like a king, lunch like a prince, and dinner like a pauper'. Avoid bad carbohydrates, like wheat and rice, after 7 p.m. Go for something light—like salads, juices, and vegetables—at night. This is really important as our body's metabolism drops down by 50 per cent at night. So if you eat heavy at night, it will be accumulated in our body as fat. Do not sleep immediately after having dinner. Sleep at least two hours later. Digest your food by taking a walk after dinner. All this won't happen immediately. It requires practice, dedication, commitment, and hard work.

I have observed many people take a new year's resolution, to be honest, towards their workout and health. They regularly do their workouts and eat healthy. As days pass by, their resolution dwindles. They lose interest, and slowly they disappear from the fitness circuit. They take a huge gap. Again one fine day, they wake up after getting stimulated by some actress's body or their friend's body, and they again join back. Now they find it tough to cope and go back to the rhythm. Finally, they struggle and give up and say it's not their cup of tea.

I would recommend to such people to do slowly and steadily whatever you can do daily even if it's for half an hour at least. This way, you will be in a continuous flow and rhythm. Don't take gaps even if you feel lazy.

I have also seen some members who suddenly disappear from the health scenario and exercise once in a blue moon in one or two months.

They state that they are too busy to work out. These same people, you will find them whiling away time in lots of useless activities. Hence, lack of time is strictly not an excuse for not working out. It's just that they are not motivated to do so.

In fact, I remember going to a society as a fitness trainer. The society was upmarket and high class. They had a gymnasium, swimming pool, squash court, and yoga studio in their health club. Plus, the management also organized group activities for the fitness class—e.g. yoga, dance—free of cost for members.

But surprisingly, very few members availed of this benefit. Hardly any members would make use of the gym and the pool. Also, the group fitness class was slowly and gradually becoming scarce with few members attending them. I would get so frustrated at them and would also curse them, saying that these members had no value for all this as they got everything free in life and at their doorstep. In spite of me encouraging and motivating them to go to the fitness group classes, very few actually turned up and were regularly attending them.

On the contrary, I remember the days when I wanted to lose weight badly. I did not have a health club in my society. I spent lakhs of rupees to be a member of India's leading gymnasiums. I used to go back and forth daily to my workout gym from my house, work, etc. Not a single day did I miss my health workout. Let me tell you, I did this along with working and taking care of my family. Such is my dedication towards fitness.

Even today, for six days a week, I indulge for a minimum of two hours of exercise daily in a mixture of cardio, yoga, dancing, and weight training. I eat healthy every day. I do allow myself a cheat day once a week, but that's it. Due to this, I reap the benefits. I am forty-seven kilograms at a height of five feet three inches. My vitals are 34, 26, 36. I have very high energy levels and, hence, able to do multitasking with ease. I am very productive at work and have good relationships. I look younger, beautiful, and totally fit. I am successful in my work.

Many of my friends ask me why am I exercising now as I don't require it. But I tell them it's just not about losing weight but about overall fitness.

In fact, they try to show off to regular members that they become too busy inducing an inferiority complex in those people who regularly do their workouts as if they don't have work and hence have the luxury to find time for workouts. I recommend that you avoid such people as they themselves don't exercise as well as demotivate those who do them. Give them a deaf ear.

Fitness is a religion to be followed daily.

Law of Attraction

You are what you think. This law is very important. In fact, you can attract all good things in your life through your thoughts. Hence, if you really want to be fit, healthy, and slim, imagine yourself to be like that. Do autosuggestions to your own self.

Those who want to be slim, please keep a role model in front of yourself. Imagine yourself to be your role model, and slowly, steadily, you will start incorporating traits of them. You will be like them. Hence, when you are working out, think of them. You will get the desired results.

Health is a never-ending discussion. It can go on and on. So many examples can be cited. So many new workouts have come out. New gyms, new yoga studios, dance classes, aerobics have started. New workouts—like aqua Zumba, hot yoga, netra yoga, aqua yoga, new dance forms—are being promoted as fitness forms.

The best part is, there is a lot of awareness and promotion of living healthy as people have understood that. Especially after 21 July has been promoted as International Yoga Day, a number of enquiries for yoga have increased ten times.

People are eating healthy. They are eating less of junk food and going slow on alcohol and smoking. In fact, in schools and colleges, children are given health education. Newspapers are devoting a section of their paper to health education. They talk about healthy food, different exercises. The whole idea is to create a health revolution. So many gyms, exercise centres, yoga centres, and dance centres have sprouted up in the last few years.

Most of the housing societies have their health clubs, gymnasiums, yoga studios, and swimming pools.

In fact, a major change has taken place even in the corporate world. Most of the companies are organizing health seminars, workshops, or yoga classes in their campuses. There are innumerable health education videos available on the Net, on Youtube. Also, there are plenty of information on health available on the Internet.

You can google it out. There are so many books available on health, nutrition, yoga, mental health, spiritual health. There are plenty of CDs available on yoga, dance as a fitness form, nutrition, etc.

Even a simple walk can change your life. So, friends, don't give this lame excuse that you don't have time. Time has to be set aside for fitness activities. Don't give another excuse that you cannot afford gym or club membership or trainers or fitness classes.

As told to you before, there are plenty of free workouts you can do, like walking, jogging. Plus, you can do that at home using the Internet, books, etc.

Where there is a will, there is a *way*. All you need is determination and dedication. So gear up and make a resolution to start your exercises today. Start eating healthy food.

Be true to yourself. Don't cheat. Be regular and sincere. Initially, it's tough, but later on, it becomes a habit. You will love it and will miss it.

My mission is to impact billions of people on this planet to improve their health and to lead a healthy, fit, disease-free life and, in the end, a happy, prosperous, and fulfilling life. They should achieve all their goals professionally and personally by this year's end.

Partly through this book, my goal will be achieved. But it will be materialized only when all of you actively do what I have preached in the book.

Thank you so much.

About the Author

Priya Chavan is a multitalented and multifaceted achiever from the financial and commercial capital of India—Mumbai. She is the founder of Priya's Wellness Center.

She is a successful entrepreneur, a distinguished academician, a corporate honcho, a talented dancer, a motivational speaker, a fitness expert, a nutritionist, a model, and an author.

She is born in a middle-class, conservative Maharashtrian family from Mumbai as one among four daughters. Her family is extremely academics oriented and only encouraged their daughters to become doctors and engineers.

She excelled academically, securing 89 per cent in SSC and 91 per cent in HSC from University of Mumbai. She did her bachelor's degree in pharmacy from India's reputed pharmacy college Bombay College of Pharmacy. In Mumbai she did her master's degree in business administration (i.e. MBA) in marketing, topping with flying colours.

She joined the corporate world in marketing in the pharmaceutical industry. She raced up the corporate ladder in multinational companies to become marketing manager.

She started her own fitness centre, Priya's Wellness, in a prime suburb in Mumbai. She faced a lot of resistance and criticism from her orthodox family for her decision to quit a high-paying job to do business which is uncertain and start from scratch. Yet she only listened to her inner call, which she had ignored for a long time, and gave a deaf ear to others.

Without any support from anyone, she started her own venture, using her own savings, skills, passion, hard work, and dynamism.

She is a first-generation entrepreneur. Her centre has trained lakhs of people of all ages worldwide in fitness groups ranging from yoga, dance as a fitness form, nutrition, meditation, functional training, kick-boxing. She leads a team of trainers under her able leadership.

She is also actively involved in conducting seminars/workshops on health, entrepreneurship, law of attraction, yoga, nutrition, dance, millionaire mindset, and success mindset in corporations as well as on individual sessions, spreading the message of good health and success.

She attributes her love of fitness to a remarkable achievement of losing twenty-five kilograms in a year's time. In that journey of weight loss, which involved intense hard work, dedication, discipline in terms of exercise, and eating healthy, she fell in love with fitness. She continues to upgrade her knowledge even now.

She is a born dancer. Besides being a Nritya Visharad in classical Kathak from Gandharva Mahavidyalaya, she also likes Western, Bollywood, Zumba, and folk dances.

She herself leads a disciplined lifestyle, exercising intensely for three hours every day, eating healthy and nutritious food, and thinking positive.

She is a powerhouse of energy. From a quiet, shy, reserved girl in her school days, she has gone a long way to become a fiery, ambitious, dynamite achiever.

She has decided to impact the health of millions of people globally through this book and her own channel of fitness Priya's Fitness Channel on Youtube.

She is a powerful leader, believing in creating leaders under her. She is extremely innovative, self-motivated, and results oriented.

She dreams big. She motivates herself by reading biographies of achievers in all walks of life—entrepreneurs like Bill Gates and Warren Buffet, sportsmen like Sachin Tendulkar, artists, dancers, singers, philosophers, writers, poets, dramatists, politicians, leaders.

She learns from them. She also reads a lot of self-development books and listens/watches videos/tapes of achievers and attends motivational seminars.

She is a very good time manager and an expert in organizing and planning. She is adventurous and takes calculated risks. She does not believe in age. She feels age is just a number. You can achieve anything in any age if you want to. If you desire something strongly from your heart, the entire universe will conspire to help you.

She has set for herself a commitment to look younger, more beautiful, and sexier with time. She is eyeing overseas locations for expansion and growth.

She has been acknowledged and recognized for her splendid work on wellness by *Corporate India*, a leading financial magazine in India.

Her inspirational story of achievement has been covered in a global portal of lady entrepreneurs: www.wearethecity.in.

She has also been recognized as a multifaceted achiever in a globally renowned e-magazine by the name of *Inspirational Unlimited*, which is the number one inspirational magazine on the Web. It is followed by readers in 115 countries and has contributing authors from more than fifty countries. The magazine has felicitated her for her wonderful contribution to improving health of lakhs of people worldwide through her venture, Priya's Wellness.

Click on the following link:

http://www.iuemag.com/september2015/is/multi-faceted-achiever.php.

To top all this, she has decided to pen down her memories in her book *My Incredible Journey*.

Her vision is to improve the health of billions of people on this planet by having 100 branches of Priya's Wellness Centre worldwide. Also, she intends to reach and create awareness among lakhs of people in India and globally by doing seminars/workshops.

To contact her, please mail her at pcpriya50@gmail.com or call 9619285427. She is available on Facebook also by the name Priya Chavan.

Printed in Dunstable, United Kingdom

77839804R00037